MS Chair Yoga
At Home

Your Step-by-Step Guide

25 Poses to Alleviate Tension, Tightness, and
Anxiety So You Can Thrive

Paula Strupeck Gardner
M.A., M.A., YACEP

ISBN: 978-1-7352276-0-3 (paperback)

Cheers to you for doing your yoga practice at home!

Thank you for purchasing, reading, and USING this book!

To receive your FREE video to practice along with me, go to:
https://awacbff.awcb.page/MS-Chair-Yoga

I'm donating 20% of net profits from this book to the MS Society, MS Focus, and other local MS groups.

* * *

If you'd like to donate directly to a particular organization, please go to:

MS Society's South Cook Self-Help Group
https://bit.ly/32DOgcW

MS Focus
https://msfocus.org/MS-Chair-Yoga-At-Home.aspx

Working on Wellness Foundation
https://www.workingonwellnessfoundation.org/

Dedicated to the Members of the MS Yoga Class at Orland Park Health and Fitness:

You inspire me and countless others.

May your journey continue to bring you peace, joy, happiness, and health.

Contents

Note From the Author

"Thank you for showing me how I can do yoga and how yoga can help me feel better—more peaceful, more focused, more comfortable...no matter what."

—From SA, longtime MS Yoga participant

Everybody can do yoga.

If you're breathing, you can do yoga.

But NOT every body can get up and down from the floor to do the traditional versions of the yoga poses.

Are you one of these people? You've heard friends talk about how great they feel after yoga—how relaxed, calm, stretched, soothed, lengthened, strengthened— but you aren't able to get down on the floor and then back up.

So how can YOUR body enjoy the benefits of yoga?

In 2003, I created chair yoga classes for my students with Multiple Sclerosis (MS), Parkinson's, COPD, arthritis, and other conditions or injuries that inhibited their ability to get up and down from the floor with ease. I used the traditional poses as inspiration but adapted them to what my students could do.

I encouraged and still encourage them to practice at least one pose each day at home and they, in turn, asked me to draw pictures of and give them descriptions of the poses to help them remember. They've been asking for a book since we began working together—a step-by-step guide to what we now call MS Chair Yoga.

THIS is the book they've been asking for—a step-by-step guide to 25 poses that my students have told me have changed their lives. Because of COVID-19, in-person classes were suspended and I've been leading them online. This nudged me to get this book into their hands and yours so you could enjoy yoga at home.

This book helps you build each pose from the ground up. It helps you put the poses together, do them with friends and family or by yourself.

- Get a free video of a guided practice that includes some of the poses in this book when you go to my site: https://awacbff.aweb.page/ MS-Chair-Yoga.

- See the poses on and do them with me as you watch my YouTube channel: https://www.youtube.com/c/MSYogaWithPaula

- Subscribe! The DVD is coming and if I have your email address, you'll be notified as soon as it's available.

- In the meantime, please join my Facebook group (https://www.facebook.com/MSYoga WithPaula) where I regularly post poses, inspiration, information and where I'll let you know about future developments.

Remember:

You're worth the work.

Everything you do counts.

As a Warrior, you exercise your courage so you can cultivate your strength.

Breathe.

Blessings Always,

Paula

Welcome!
Here's How to Use This Book and Why

I've been teaching long enough to know that you're likely to use this book in the way(s) that is unique to you. Some of you will simply open to the page you want to look at. Others will read it cover to cover 4 times before you do any of it. Still others of you will take it pose by pose and try each before you move on. You'll each do what you want. And this is good!

With that in mind, I'd **love** for you to start here before you go to wherever it is you're going.

It will be helpful to you to read **my philosophy** so that you know what the heck I'm talking about and where I'm coming from and how you can use it to build and enhance your yoga.

It will also be helpful to you to read the **guiding principles of a successful yoga practice**. Successful means you get out of it what you want. We want it to be safe. We want your yoga practice to fit with your life. And **I** want you to do yoga for the rest of your life.

I'm not a doctor. I make no claims for instantaneous (or ANY) remission of the multiple sclerosis. What I offer is a proven way to help you live your life with vibrancy and a way to reduce or eliminate some of your aches and pains (inner and outer!). "Proven" in that I've been sharing yoga with the group of folks (whose comments are sprinkled throughout this book) for over 15 years and they report and I observe how gracefully they live with this disease, how supportive they are of each other, and how yoga has helped them on their journey—keeping them as limber of mind/body/spirit as they can be, engaging with their loved ones and their not-so-loved ones, meeting life with an equanimity that I envy.

You can have this too. Use this book to help you get there.

Each pose has its own page with an in-depth description of how to get into, hold, and then out of the pose. And a photo to guide you as well.

At the end of the book, you'll find a couple of sequences (poses grouped together with an intention in mind) that you can practice. I invite you to subscribe to my YouTube channel (https://www. youtube.com/c/MSYogaWithPaula) so that you can SEE the poses in action and hear me talk you through them. To be notified of updates and future videos and books, subscribe to my email at this site—https://awacbff.aweb.page/MS-Chair-Yoga.

As always, remember:

Breathe deeply in and even more deeply out.
Let the breath come to you.

You're worth the work. And the play!

Namaste.

P.S. The model for all of the photos in this book is my long-time yoga student (though I believe I've learned far more from her than the other way around) Anne Matty. For all of the years that we were together, creating and tweaking and playing with the poses, Anne was a stalwart supporter of everyone, teacher included, who entered our sacred yoga space. She was, until she moved to be near her grandchildren, everyone's Mom. The program at OPHFC remains strong, but the gaping hole that her departure left will not be filled. I am forever grateful to her for her time and her devotion to her "yoga kids."

"When I first began yoga classes, I hated them. I thought it was a waste of time. The more I attended classes, the more comfortable I felt with the different poses, stretches, and turns. I'm almost at the point where I look forward to going. And this is a huge compliment to you, Paula."

—SLA, longtime MS Yoga participant

My Philosophy
Yoga is About You

As you begin yoga or as you use this book to expand and strengthen your yoga connection, it's important to me that you know how and why I advocate what I do. This knowledge, I believe, will help you trust me. And trust—of yourself, the process, the teacher—is really important to your lifelong yoga journey. So, I share with you my "philosophy of yoga." As you use the poses to live your intention (strength, flexibility, focus, peace of mind, relaxation...), it will help you to understand where I'm coming from.

Yoga is about YOU. It's not about the poses. Or perfect form. Or perfect anything.

Having been trained by teachers who were Iyengar-trained or heavily influenced by BKS Iyengar's alignment focus and philosophy of bringing the pose to the person rather than forcing the person into the pose, I put a lot of energy into figuring out ways to make yoga poses accessible to those who do yoga seated in a chair or have physical limitations.

"Let the pose be a manifestation of YOU rather than you manifesting the pose" is what I regularly repeat to all my students.

If you are breathing, you can do yoga.

I believe this all the way down to my toes. The changes, the growth, the peace, the joy that yoga has led me to over the course of 20+ years of practice and teaching are beyond counting. In yoga poses, we make space in the body for the breath. In doing this, we learn to make space in our life for our self.

The simplest, most straightforward version of a pose done with attention to breath and awareness of body opens our body, heart and mind in ways that the most complex or advanced version done with inattention or unawareness cannot.

For you who have MS, Parkinson's or other illnesses that affect your ability to move, I recommend following the advice of Dr. Loren Fishman and Eric Small, a yoga practitioner who sought out yoga to help him stay healthy when he was diagnosed at age 22 with MS. (He's now in his 80's.) Hold the active poses for up to 3 breaths. No more. Restorative poses are treated differently. I note in the pose descriptions how long it's recommended to hold the pose.

It is awareness, after all, that creates our yoga.

No matter whether we sit or stand or lie down, our awareness determines our level of participation and our progress in the practice. When we desire strength or flexibility or focus or relaxation, we must know what we have, how we do things, and where we stand RIGHT NOW or we're limited in how we can create and expand this strength, flexibility, focus, or relaxation. We must be aware of our breathing patterns in order to manage our breath. We must be aware of how we sit in order to sit more healthfully. We must be aware of where our knees and feet are in order to move them to a position that's better for our body.

Awareness leads us to create greater health of mind, body, spirit.

In Ayurveda, the sister science of yoga (the ancient Eastern approach to health and well-being) mind, body, and spirit are considered one and inseparable. What we do for or to one, we do for or to the others. So it behooves us to breathe and move with awareness, to place our limbs in positions that are healthy and intentional rather than random. And when the body doesn't/can't cooperate, we must use the mind to instruct, encourage, create.

Many, MANY studies in recent years have demonstrated the incredible connection between mind and body. The study I love to cite but can't find the source for was done with baseball players where the athletes wore devices that measured the electro-magnetic activity in their muscles while they were performing their game tasks—throwing, catching, running, batting. The athletes were then taken into a lab, taught relaxation for 10 minutes then instructed to visualize their game activities—throwing, catching, running, batting. The muscle activity was then remeasured and found to be THE SAME AS WHEN THEY WERE ACTUALLY PERFORMING.

This is how strong the mind-body connection is.

MS might inhibit the ability to move exactly as you want, but when you visualize, you acknowledge and feed this powerful connection of mind and body. You inform the body that this is the direction you want to go. I can't prove to you with any degree of statistical power that this will happen for you, but I know that our mind/body connection is immeasurably powerful and that in honoring this connection, you sustain and thrive in the face of this ravaging disease.

Intention gives direction to awareness.

At the beginning of each class, I invite participants to ask themselves why they came to yoga on this day. And to choose JUST ONE of these things to become their intention for the day's practice...or maybe for the day! The intention gives direction to your awareness, allows you to do each pose with a focus that allows the mind/body to participate fully in the process and helps them receive the benefits of this day's yoga.

We all do the best we know how.

Many years ago, I had the privilege of working with a blind man who shared this bit of wisdom with me: "We all do the best we know how." At any given moment, on any given day, we're able to do things... or not. I encourage you to accept the body you're in, not the one you always wanted, not the one you had 20 years ago, but the one you're in today. Accepting where we are, the body we're in, what we can do at this moment allows us to be present and to move more freely than when we are caught in the web of what "I used to be able to do" or "what I want to do." At the same time, when we're feeling bad about where we are and we acknowledge this feeling, we're able to move with and beyond it.

I love the image of our emotions being like a cloud being blown across the sky until it's out of our sight. The emotions hang around only as long as we hold onto them.

I never said it was easy.

And *you're worth the work.*

It's a lot to think about and do all at the same time. We line up the bones so that muscles don't have to work as hard, but lining up the bones and lining up our minds and emotions all at the same time is challenging. And focusing on the breath. And letting go of judgment, shame, criticism, despair, frustration. And listening to instructions. And working to create a pose with a body part that doesn't work as it once did. All at the same time. Yikes!

Receive the breath. Breathe deeply in. Breathe even more deeply out.

And remind yourself: You're worth the work.

And the play. Remember to play.

> *"Paula is able to adjust the poses for our different disabilities..."*

—From AM, longtime MS Yoga participant

> *"Over the years, Paula has been an invaluable and trusted resource in my continued efforts to improve my health and well-being. I've benefitted not only from her knowledge, but also from her inspiration, wisdom and kindness. In such a fast-paced world, Paula takes the time to truly listen and understand your needs and work with you to accomplish what you set out to do.*

She offers just the right level of the patience and gentle nudging so necessary to keep a person on the track to success."

—AYJ, longtime yoga participant

"I don't know what I'd do without Paula in my life. She is truly a wonderful, giving person."

—AMM, Long-time MS Yoga participant

Guiding Principles of a Successful Yoga Practice or The KISS of Chair Yoga

1.*Awareness is key.* You start unaware or with a limited awareness of your body and how it moves and you grow with your practice. Start with your breath and move from there. (See #8.)

2.*Wear comfortable clothing that moves with you.* If something is too baggy, it will get in your way. If something is too tight or the fabric doesn't move, it will impair your ability to move.

3.*Don't just sit there.* If you can't do something, visualize yourself doing it. Your muscles get the message that this is where you want them to head. The mind/body connection is amazingly and incredibly strong. But it starts in and with you. Remember, you're "moving in the direction of..."

4.*Be kind to yourself.* Have you ever done yoga before? I never said it would be easy. Have you done yoga in the past and you're frustrated because your body isn't doing what it used to do? Have you been doing yoga and you're noticing changes in how your body is responding? Have you been doing yoga and today just feels different? It all counts. You're worth your awareness. You're worth your attention. Remember: we all do the best we can do at any given moment on any given day.

5.*Get SOFT*. Contrary to popular opinion, yoga is more about softening (in my book!) than it is about stretching. Stretching is work and challenges and tightens the muscles. You do (we all do) enough of this kind of work everywhere else in our life. While you're doing yoga, focus your awareness and intention on SOFTENING. You'll find that this carries over into other parts of your life and you'll feel better for it. You may experience less fatigue because you're releasing even more tension. It's work to let go. You're worth the work.

6.*If there's PAIN, there is NO GAIN*. A critical part of experiencing yoga is learning to discern discomfort from pain. Discomfort tells us we're doing something differently than we're used to doing. This is often a good thing because we're learning to do things in a more healthful way. PAIN is never good except as a messenger that we need to STOP what we're doing and pay attention. And do it differently or not at all.

7.*Commit to yourself and to the process*. Doing one yoga pose each day is more desirable than doing an hour of poses once a month or even once a week. Plus, the Kaizen method teaches us that when we do only one thing, the limbic brain doesn't put up resistance or induce anxiety as thinking of 30 minutes of yoga does. It all counts. One is a great beginning.

8.*Let your breath lead your movement.* Begin to breathe in and THEN begin to move. Begin to breathe out and THEN begin to move. When your awareness drifts, everything drifts.

The Poses We Do

Following is a list of the poses that are described and pictured in this book.

Each pose is, on subsequent pages, described in detail about where to place the body, how to sit on the chair as this applies, things to pay attention to in the poses and things to pay attention to as you get into and out of the pose. A photograph accompanies each pose to give you the overall idea of where you're headed.

Following the descriptions of the poses, you'll find a couple of practices—ways in which to organize the poses for your at-home yoga practice. Keep in mind that, as you become more and more familiar with the poses, you'll be able to listen to your body and intuit what would make the most sense for you on any given day.

You can practice the poses with me when you go to my YouTube channel (https://www.youtube.com/c/MSYogaWithPaula). To receive updates about videos and books and to get a free video of an active chair yoga practice, type your name and email address at this site: https://awacbff.aweb.page/MS-Chair-Yoga.

List of Our Chair Yoga Poses

- Seated Tadasana Sitting isn't just sitting: It's sitting with awareness.

- Cat/Cow (Bidalasana)

- Cobbler's Pose (Baddha konasana)

- Cow Face Arms

- Eagle Arms

- Extended Seated Angle

- Finger/Hand/Shoulder Release

- Forward Fold

- Half Easy-Sitting Pose or #4 Pose (Ardha Sukhasana)

- Interlacing Fingers

- Knot

- Psoas Softener and Toner

- Shoulder Circles

- Side Stretch

- Standing Tadasana

- Sun Salutation

- Supported Forward Fold

- Top of Hand Stretch

- Twist One

- Twist Two

- Twist Three

- Warrior 1 and 2 (Virabhadrasana 1 and 2)

- Wide-legged Tadasana

- Savasana (Final Relaxation)

Step by Step Guide to Each Pose

The poses are listed in alphabetical order after Seated Mountain (Tadasana) to make it easier for you to find them on your own. The reason I've placed Seated Tadasana first is that it is the foundation for each seated pose. The reason I've placed Savasana (Final

Relaxation) at the end is that each practice needs to end with at least a few minutes of sitting peacefully, letting your mind/body/spirit absorb the poses and the residual effects on your central nervous system.

Please note that it's important to begin each practice whether it's 1 pose or 10 poses by sitting in Tadasana and centering your mind and your awareness on what you're going to do next.

In our classes, we begin by scanning the body from the head to the toes and feeling for where we feel strong and where we could use a little help that day. Next, we listen to the breath and feel where we feel the breath coming into the body (nose or mouth), where we feel the breath once it's in the body (chest? belly? sides? back?) and then where we feel it leaving the body (nose or mouth).

Starting out with awareness makes it easier to bring awareness to how we feel in each pose.

For the poses where you need more than the chair you're sitting in (and the blocks under your feet IF you need them), the additional props (blocks, chair, strap and/or bolster/sofa cushion) are listed before the instructions.

I've included a helpful hint after some of the poses. These are things that I've shared in classes that my students have said have helped them find and experience the pose. I trust you will too!

Let's begin! Let's do some yoga!

Seated Mountain (Tadasana)

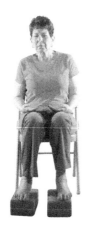 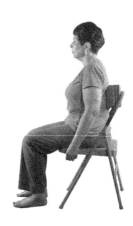

You need only one chair. You MAY need a block or 3 depending on your height and if you want or need support behind you. (You may also use a stiff pillow or cushion behind you for support.) (See resources for information on purchasing blocks and a strap.)

Sitting isn't just sitting. It's sitting with awareness.

Sit away from the back of your chair. Do NOT lean against the back of your chair. When we lean against our chair, our back rounds, our shoulders round and our chest caves in. This means we're inhibiting deep breathing. We're cutting off our ability to take in breath. We're also causing our spine to round where it's not meant to. For support, you can place a block between you and the chair at your shoulder blades. If your feet are not flat on the floor, use one block under each foot.

Line up your knees with your hips and your knees over your ankles. Look at your feet. Place your feet so that the outer edges and the big toes are parallel with each other, with the walls or with your mat if you're using a mat.

Many people stand and walk like ducks with our toes pointing out to varying degrees.

We want to practice sitting and standing with our feet in a healthier position (outer edges and big toes parallel to the walls) so that it becomes something we do when we're not practicing yoga. We want to create new neural pathways so that we position our feet in the healthiest way possible when we're walking around.

As you sit, lift your heart and feel for the curve in your lower back. Keep your heart lifting and draw your lowest ribs into your body so that they're level with the front of your pelvis. The first 1000 times, you may want to use your hands to gently guide your ribs in since this may be an action you're not used to doing.

The reason to draw your lowest ribs in is that it engages your core muscles. In fact, when you do this over time, you'll begin to notice a sensation of engaging or a slight tightening deep in your abdomen.

This is good!

Relax your hands on your thighs. Line up your nose with your chin with your belly button.

I encourage you to close your eyes. When we close our eyes, we're signaling to the parasympathetic nervous system to run instead of the sympathetic nervous system. We pretty much live in the sympathetic nervous system—fight or flight or freeze.

We need every day to spend 20 minutes (twice a day if you can do it) in a position that allows the parasympathetic nervous system to work in order to take the body out of operating in the sympathetic nervous system. Dr. Herbert Benson discovered and wrote about what he called the Relaxation Response in 1975. Since then, lots of research has discussed how important accessing our parasympathetic nervous system is to our health.

Helpful hint: You could stay here and breathe, focusing on your breath, a prayer, a peaceful word for 20 minutes and reap great benefits from your time here.

Tadasana is the foundation of all poses.

Cat/Cow

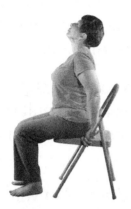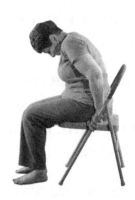

The tricky part of doing these two poses is that we tend to move back and forth in our chair. This is NOT what we want. Instead, keep your shoulders over your hips and let only your spine move into an arch and then into a rounded back. When you do this regularly, you may well notice that you have greater mobility in your spine.

Begin in Tadasana. Hold onto the sides of the seat.

Begin to inhale and lift your heart forward and your chin up a little. Arch your back.

Begin to exhale and begin rounding your back toward, letting your head hang forward and down.

Remember keep your shoulders over your hips.

You may also find it helpful to do the poses the following way:

> Place your hands on your knees so that your fingertips are below your knee caps and the heel of your hands is above your knee caps.
>
> Begin to inhale and press your fingertips into your legs below your kneecaps and pull your heart forward, lifting your chest and your chin and your gaze up.
>
> Begin to exhale and press the heel of your hands into your legs above your kneecaps and press your back toward the chair, letting it round and letting your head hang.

Helpful hint: Remember to keep your shoulders over your hips. The idea is to stay upright and not to move forward and back over your thighs.

Helpful hint: Practice initiating the movement at your pelvis. When you inhale, tilt the top of your pelvis forward. When you exhale, tilt the top of your pelvis back.

Cobbler's Pose (Baddha Konasana) Versions 1 & 2

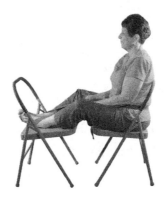

Anne is pictured in version 1

You'll need 2 chairs and 1 strap OR 1 chair, 1 strap and 2 blocks (You may enjoy having a block or a thick cushion behind your back.)

Version 1

Begin in Tadasana.

Sit on your chair with the seat of a second chair facing you.

Place your feet on the seat of the chair opposite you and bring your strap around the pinkie toe sides of your feet. Hold onto the strap and gently pull your feet in toward you. Remember, if there's pain there is no gain so only do a little at a time.

Lift your heart and draw your lowest ribs in to be even with the top of your pelvis.

Stay here for a few breaths in and out.

To come out of the pose, release the strap from around your feet and place one foot down to the floor and then the other.

If you are unable to lift your feet to the seat of a chair in front of you, use version 2.

Version 2

Begin in Tadasana.

Sit on your chair and place 2 blocks on the floor at whatever height works for you. Rest the pinkie toe sides of your feet on the blocks. You may find that it helps to bring the strap around that sides of your feet or you may like it better without the strap in this position. Choose what works for you.

Sit up straight and tall. Lift your heart, draw your lowest ribs in to be even with the top of your pelvis.

Stay here for a few breaths in and out.

Helpful hint: As you stay in the pose, I encourage you to visualize any part of your body that feels tense or tight, one at a time. When you bring awareness to a body part, that body part responds by softening and relaxing.

Cow Face Arms

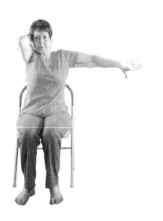 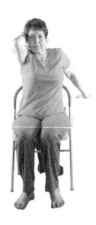

Begin in Tadasana pose with your feet flat on the floor or on blocks as you need. (You may want to hold a necktie or a yoga strap in your upper hand to begin. This is optional.)

Sit facing forward in the center of your chair.

Bend your right elbow so that it's pointing forward and your fingertips touch your right shoulder. If you can lift your elbow higher without it going outward, feel free to lift it higher. Remember to let it do what it can do and NOT force it into where you want it to be.

Stretch your left arm straight out to the left side, thumb down.

Inhale. Begin exhaling and reach the left hand back back back and back...as far back as you can get and THEN bend your left elbow and rest your hand against your back or the back of your chair. Some people like to hold a strap while they hold this position.

Breathe three breaths in and out. Release your hands and arms down.

Do the other side:

> Bend your left elbow so that it's pointing forward and your fingertips touch your left shoulder. If you can lift your elbow higher without it going outward, feel free to lift it higher. Remember to let it do what it can do and not force it into where you want it to be.

> Stretch your right arm straight out to the right side, thumb down.

> Inhale. Begin exhaling and reach the right hand back back back and back...as far back as you can get and THEN bend your right elbow and rest your hand against your back or the back of your chair.

Breathe three breaths in and out. Release your hands and arms down.

Eagle Arms

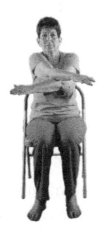 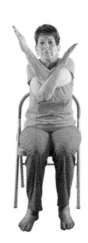

Begin in Tadasana.

Begin inhaling and stretch your arms out into a T, keeping your hands slightly below your shoulder height.

Begin exhaling and bring your arms forward to cross the right arm over the left at the elbows if you can manage or your forearms if you cannot cross at the elbows.

If your arms are crossed at the forearms, on your next exhale reach your fingertips forward.

IF your arms are crossed at the elbows, on your next exhale, bend your elbows with the backs of your hands facing each other. They don't have to touch. Don't try to make them touch. When your shoulders are open enough, the backs of your hands will be closer together. It is NOT our goal to touch the backs of our hands in this pose. Our goal is to HONOR what the body can do right now.

Hold for 3 breaths. On the 4th inhale, sweep your arms out to the sides as though you're an eagle spreading your wings.

Repeat with the left arm over the right arm.

Helpful hint: Since the purpose of this pose is to relax and release the shoulder blades and shoulders, there is no point in striving to get the backs of the hands together. Let the body open at its pace and on its time table.

Extended Side Angle

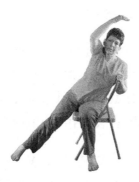

Begin in Tadasana.

Turn to the right and sit sideways in your chair. Sit so that the back of your right knee is touching the seat of the chair. If you have blocks under your feet to bring the floor to you, place one under your right foot as you sit sideways.

Begin inhaling and stretch your arms up to the sky.

Begin exhaling and lean over the back of your chair so that your armpit is resting on the top of the back of the chair and your left arm stretches over your head. Face the palm down.

Stretch your left leg out to the side and point your toes to the right.

Visualize your breath moving the entire length of your left side, from your heel along your leg, up your side body, along your arm out through your finger tips.

Breathe 3 slow, long, even, deep breaths in and 3 slow long even deep breaths out.

On your 4th inhale, reach your left arm up to the sky. As you exhale, bring that arm under your left thigh and help your thigh forward so that your knees are even and your whole body is facing to the right again.

Come back to the center of your chair to sit in Tadasana for a breath in and a breath out.

Then do the other side.

Helpful hint: This is one of the very few times that you will notice I'm saying lean against the back of your chair. Take advantage of it!

Finger/Hand/Shoulder Release

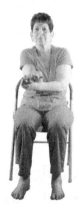

Version 1

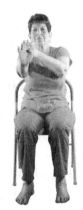

Version 2

Begin in Tadasana.

This pose has two versions. Please choose the one that best fits your body. If you're able to hold your arms straight out in front of you, choose version 2. If you can't straighten and keep your arms straight, choose version 1.

Version 1

Bend your elbows and face your palms up.

Start with the right hand.

Bring the left hand under the right hand and place your index (pointer) finger on top of the middle of your right thumb. Inhale. Begin exhaling and gently pull the thumb down towards your lap.

Begin inhaling and move your left index finger to the right index finger's middle knuckle (You're still under the right hand.). Begin exhaling and gently pull the index finger down.

Begin inhaling and move your left index finger to the middle knuckle of the middle finger of the right hand. Begin exhaling and gently pull the middle finger down.

Begin inhaling and move your left index finger to the middle knuckle of the ring (4th) finger of your right hand. Begin exhaling and gently pull the ring finger down.

Being inhaling and move your left index finger to the middle knuckle of the pinkie (5th) finger of your right hand. Begin exhaling and gently pull the pinkie finger down.

Begin inhaling and move your left index finger back to the middle knuckle of your right thumb. Begin exhaling and gently pull the thumb down and hold it down for 3 slow long even deep breaths in and out.

Relax both hands to your lap. You may want to shake your hands out a bit before moving to the opposite side.

Helpful hint: Remember to continue to face the palm of your hand upwards and to pull from under the hand.

Version 2

Stretch your arms straight out in front of you. Keep your hands just below shoulder height.

Keep facing the palms forward.

Begin inhaling and bring the index finger of your right hand to the underside of the middle of your left thumb. Begin exhaling and gently pull the thumb toward you, keeping the palm facing forward.

Begin inhaling and bring the index finger of your right hand to the underside of the middle of your left index finger. Begin exhaling and gently pull the finger toward you.

Begin inhaling and bring the index finger of your right hand to the underside of the middle of your left middle finger. Begin exhaling and gently pull the finger toward you.

Begin inhaling and bring the index finger of your right hand to the underside of the middle of your left ring (4th) finger. Begin exhaling and gently pull the finger toward you.

Begin inhaling and bring the index finger of your right hand to the underside of the middle of your left pinkie (5th) finger. Begin exhaling and gently pull the finger toward you.

Begin inhaling and bring the index finger of your right hand back to the underside of the middle of your left thumb. Begin exhaling and gently pull the thumb toward you. Hold your thumb toward you for 3 slow long even deep breaths in and out.

Release your hands to your lap. You may want to shake your hands out a bit before moving to the opposite side.

Helpful hint: Remember to face the palm forward.

If you can do version 2 with one hand and not the other, do whichever version feels better for each.

Forward Fold

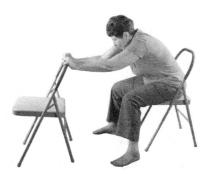

You'll need a second chair for this pose. Or you can use a wall or a table.

Begin in Tadasana.

Place the second chair directly in front of you, so that the back of the second chair faces you. It's easier if the second chair is on a surface that allows it to be pushed forward. If this isn't possible, play with the distance between the chairs until you find where you need it to be to comfortably place your hands on the top of the chair and stretch forward.

Place your hands on the top of the back of the second chair.

Inhale. Begin exhaling and allow yourself to fold forward FROM YOUR WAIST. Keep your upper back straight and keep the curve in your lower back as you fold forward.

Once you're stretched forward, draw your lowest ribs in to be level with the top of your pelvis. Then begin softening the curve in your lower back.

Pretend you're holding a giant grapefruit between your chin and your chest. This helps you keep your chin from jutting forward which scrunches the back of your neck. We want your neck to feel relaxed and long.

Inhale the breath. And exhale. Stay here for several slow, long, even, deep breaths in and out, allowing yourself to let go of tension in your shoulders, your upper back, your middle back, your lower back, your arms and your neck.

If the second chair is on a surface where it can move, push the chair forward as you stretch forward. If the chair is on a carpet or some other surface where it can't move, adjust where you put it so that you can lean forward, place your hands on the top of the back of the chair and stretch out, keeping your upper back straight.

Helpful hint: It's common to have a fair amount of tightness as well as the desire to go as far forward as you can. "Going far forward" is not the point of this pose. The point is to support the spine as you're lengthening it. So. remember to come forward from your hips and your pelvis and not your upper back. Keep the upper back straight. Keep the lower back in its healthy curve and allow it to soften as you hold the pose

Half Easy Sitting Pose or #4 Pose (Ardha Sukhasana)

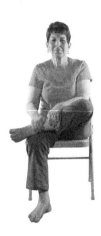

Begin in Tadasana.

Lift your right leg and place your right ankle on your left thigh.

If your right knee is really high and at an angle, I recommend that you do Wide-sitting Tadasana instead (Wide-angle Tadasana is at the end of this list). If you're comfortable with your right leg parallel to the ground, then this is your pose. You can stay here for several breaths.

While you're here, close your eyes and breathe and visualize your breath moving into and out of your right hip area. It's like you're doing spring cleaning: Each time you breathe out, your breath is sweeping away all the dust and debris that have settled here over the years from held anger, resentment, disappointment, sorrow, fear.

To come out, begin breathing in and as you breathe out, lower your right foot to the floor. Pause for several breaths before you begin the other side. AND, you may find that the other side is very different. The right side might not be able to do this pose this way, but the left side can. Or vice versa. Honor your body as it is today.

Interlacing Fingers

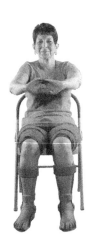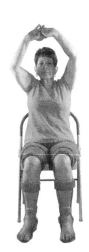

Begin in Tadasana.

Stretch your arms out in front of you. Clasp your hands together. Notice which thumb is on top. Keep your fingers intertwined and press your palms away from you. If it's accessible, reach your hands over your head, palms facing the sky. If that's not available to you, keep gently pressing your palms away from you.

Stay where you are for 3 slow long even deep breaths in and out.

At the end of the 3rd exhale, relax your hands and arms to your sides. Shake them a bit if this feels right to do.

Stretch your arms out in front of you again. Clasp your hands. Notice which thumb is on the outside. This time, rearrange your fingers and thumb so that the opposite thumb is on the outside. If it doesn't feel weird, you didn't change anything!

Keep your fingers intertwined and press your palms away from you. If it's accessible, reach your hands over your head, palms facing the sky. If that's not available to you, keep gently pressing your palms away from you.

Stay where you are for 3 slow long even deep breaths in and out.

At the end of the 3rd exhale, relax your hands and arms to your sides. Shake them a bit if this feels right to do.

Knot

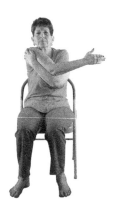

Begin in Tadasana.

Bring your right hand across your body to hold under your left armpit. Stretch the left arm across your body to the right. Inhale. Begin exhaling and reach the fingertips of your left hand to the right. Stay here for 3 slow long even deep breaths in and out.

Release your hands to your sides.

Bring your left hand across your body to hold under your right armpit. Stretch the right arm across your body to the left. Inhale. Begin exhaling and reach the fingertips of your right hand to the right. Stay here for 3 slow long even deep breaths in and out.

Helpful hint: You want to stretch but not overstretch. Let yourself feel graceful as you reach your fingertips.

"My favorite pose is being still and breathing."

—CA, Long-time MS Yoga Practitioner

Psoas Softener and Toner

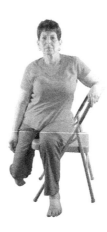

This pose, after Tadasana, may be the most important pose that you do.

The psoas (pronounced "so as") is the biggest and strongest and deepest muscle in the group of muscles called the hip flexors. It has a fairly important job: It is the only muscle that connects the legs to the spine!

But the importance of the psoas is even deeper than this. My friend Linda Troutman always says, "So as the psoas" because it plays such a critical role in our overall health and well-being as well as connecting the legs to the spine. And the rest of the body goes according to what the psoas is doing. So as the psoas goes, so goes the rest of the body.

The psoas muscles support the internal organs and help pump blood and lymph in and out of our cells. PLUS, the psoas muscles are connected to the diaphragm (our breathing muscle) via ligaments and fascia. And this is important to remember: When we get stressed, the psoas contracts. It influences and reacts to our fight or flight response.

It can be challenging to know whether your psoas is tight or too loose, but your body lets you know.

Because it's such an important muscle, it's worthwhile to do things to tone it every day.

Here's one thing you can do lying on the floor or on your bed:

Lie on your back. Bend your knees and place your feet on the floor (or bed) so they're hip distance apart and parallel to each other. Bring your heels in toward your buttocks, maybe a foot away. Now here's the hard part: Just lie here for 10-15 minutes. Let gravity do its thing. It will release tension in the psoas muscles and it will help the whole self be in a healthier state of mind/body/spirit!

Here's the pose you can do in your chair:

Begin in Tadasana.

Turn to your right. Sit sideways in the chair with the back of your right knee touching the seat of the chair (your right foot on a block if it needs to be) and your left buttock hanging off the chair. If you feel safer having a second chair at your side, please do this.

Place your right arm on the top of the back of the chair and lift your heart up and draw your lowest ribs in so they're even with the top of your pelvis.

Let your left knee point down toward the ground and rest the top of your foot on the ground or on a block. Take care to stay centered so you don't make a C with your body, leaning your shoulder toward the back of the chair.

Press your right buttock into the chair and lengthen your right side from under your arm to the seat of the chair. Bring the bottom of your pelvis slightly forward, as though you're pointing the tailbone toward the ground. When you do this, you'll notice sensation in the upper left thigh. This tells you you're in the right place.

Begin inhaling and lift your left arm straight up to the sky. Stay here for 3 breaths in and out. Then let your hand come down to your side or your lap and visualize your breath moving into and out of the space from just below your rib cage to just above your knee cap.

See if you can experience that side of your body feeling as though it's letting go of tension and tightness. You can stay here for several breathing cycles.

Helpful hint: Sometimes, the foot gets uncomfortable. You can support it with a block or a cushion under the shin which lifts the foot up a bit.

After several breaths, come back to the center of your chair for Tadasana. Pause here for a breath or two and then go to the other side.

Helpful hint: Focus on softening, not on stretching or working. Let gravity as you lie or sit take care of releasing and relaxing the muscles. You may even notice that as one muscle relaxes, that relaxation spreads to other muscles too.

"I enjoy all the poses, but I have to say my favorite one is when we soften the psoas muscle. I'm always so tight and that really helps me feel better."

—AMM long-time MS Yoga Participant

"I'm afraid I'll fall off the chair when we do this. Paula always brings a second chair in front of me so that I feel safer...She seems like she's only talking and helping me. She makes me feel so important. It feels very personalized."

—SLA, long-time MS Yoga Participant

Shoulder Circles

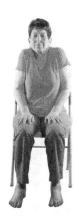

Begin in Tadasana.

Begin inhaling and lift your shoulders to your ears. Begin exhaling and move your shoulders back and down.

Begin inhaling and moving your shoulders forward and up. Begin exhaling and move your shoulders back and down.

Repeat this 3-5 times. Slowly and easily.

Side Stretch

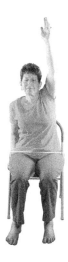

Begin in Tadasana.

Place your left hand on the seat of the chair.

Begin inhaling and lift your right arm up toward the sky, palm facing the midline of your body.

Reach your right buttock into the chair. Visualize your breath moving the full length of your right side, from your buttock up along your side body up under your arm and up the length of your arm to your hand and fingers.

Stay here for 3 slow long even deep breaths in and out. At the end of the 3rd exhale, relax your right arm down. Pause for a breath in and out.

Do the other side.

Place your right hand on the seat of the chair.

Begin inhaling and lift your left arm up toward the sky, palm facing the midline of your body.

Reach your left buttock into the chair. Visualize your breath moving the full length of your left side, from your buttock up along your side body up under your arm and up the length of your arm to your hand and fingers.

Stay here for 3 slow long even deep breaths in and out. At the end of the 3rd exhale, relax your left arm down. Pause for a breath in and out.

Standing Tadasana

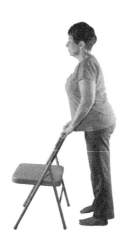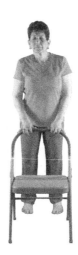

Place the chair (or your walker if you use one and feel safer with it) in front of you. Place your hands on the top of the back of the chair if you feel safer this way.

This is an active, intentional approach to standing.

Stand with your feet about hip width apart. Place your feet so that the outside edges are parallel to the walls.

Press your feet down. Press your calves out. (Imagine hands on your calves pressing in and you resist the hands and press out.) Use the muscles in the fronts of your thighs to lift your knee caps. You're not bending your knees. You're lifting the knees caps up toward your hips.

Spin your thighs in and back. (Place your hands on the outside of your thighs and gently move them forward and in and then press back.) Let your butt go with. (Now let your hands relax at your sides or rest on the top of the back of your chair.)

Lift your heart, widen your collar bones. Keep your heart lifting and draw your lowest ribs in so they're even with the front of your pelvis. Bring your chin to be parallel to the ground and lift the crown (the top) of your head up.

Helpful hint: For as long as you're standing in Tadasana, keep starting over from the bottom up. All of these things are happening at the same time as the ones before and after, so it takes a fair amount of your concentration.

You're worth it.

Practice this pose everywhere you go. Only you know you're doing it. It will help you stand and walk taller. It will help your circulation. It will help you breathe more deeply and evenly in your everyday life.

If you use a walker, take care to keep the walker close to you and to walk with your heart lifted rather than leaning over the walker.

If you are wheelchair-bound, the wide-legged tadasana is extremely important for you to do daily.

Sun Salutation (Surya Namaskar)

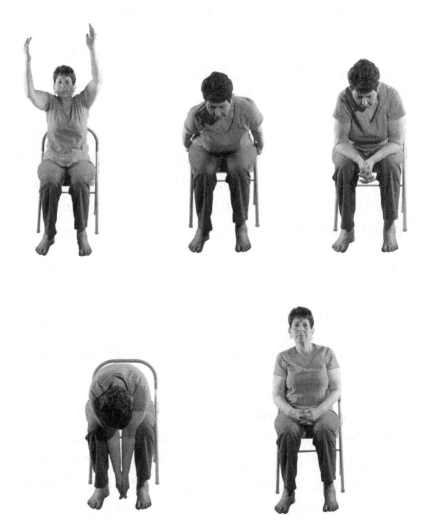

Begin in Tadasana.

Begin breathing in and lift your hands up over your head.

Begin breathing out and fold forward, with your hands behind you holding onto the back of the chair.

Straighten your arms as best you can.

Breathing in, lift your heart and spin your upper arms away from your body. (Think of the inside of your elbows as pointing forward.)

Breathing out, let go of the chair and drape yourself over your lap. If your hands will reach, place them on a block between your feet or let your fingertips touch the ground. If the ground is too far away, place your forearms on your thighs.

Wherever you go, let your head hang so that the top of your head is pointing down to the ground. Let it be heavy as a bowling ball. Breathe in and out here.

Very gently, shake your head no. Even more gently, nod your head yes.

Beginning to inhale, press your forearms into your thighs to lift your upper body just a bit. Beginning to exhale, press your feet down, press your thighs into the chair, draw your lowest ribs gently in and come up to a seated position.

Pause for a breath in and a breath out. Begin again.

Do 1-3 of these salutations to help you warm and energize the body.

Supported Forward Fold

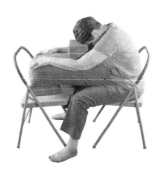

You'll need a second chair, as many as 4 blocks if you're using blocks under your feet, and a very thick and sturdy sofa cushion or a yoga bolster. And a blanket if you'd like.

You'll also need to pay great attention to how you feel because you'll need to adjust the props according to your body. The props are meant to bring the pose to you. You are not meant to go to the pose.

Anne has used one block under the bolster and one block on the bolster under her head. You can use two blocks under the bolster or two blocks on top of the bolster or you may not need the blocks at all. You might need more blocks AND the blanket. It's all good as long as you're honoring your body's need for comfort.

Play with it until it's comfortable for you. (And it may change over time.)

Face the two chairs toward each other. To follow Anne's example, place one block on the chair and the bolster on the block. Let the bolster be touching your belly.

Begin in Tadasana. Breathe the breath in and lengthen the front of your spine by lifting your heart up. Breathe out and lean forward over the bolster, supporting your head with the block on its baby bear side. (Again, you might want it higher.)

You can stay here for several minutes. As long as you're comfortable. In fact you might want to set a gentle timer for yourself so that if you really zoned out, you'll have a gentle reminder to come back!

When you're ready, breathe in and press your hands down on the bolster or the chair to lift yourself up. Give yourself a few breaths in and out to come back to reality.

Top of Hand Stretch

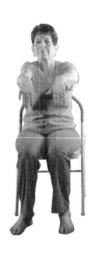 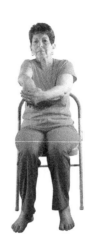

Begin in Tadasana.

Reach your arms straight out in front of you, hands just below shoulder height.

Let your right finger tips point down to the ground.

Place your left palm on the top of your right hand and gently press the top of the right hand. Hold for 3 slow long even deep breaths in and out.

Relax your hands to your lap. Pause for a breath and a breath out.

Repeat on the other side.

Twist One

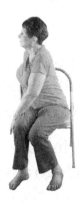

Begin in Tadasana.

Inhale the breath and reach your hands up to the sky.

Beginning to breathe out, walk your left foot and knee slightly forward, turn gently toward your right side, drawing your lowest ribs into your body. Let your hands come down, your right hand behind you; your left hand in front of you.

Stay here for 3 slow long even deep breaths in and out, mindful of drawing the lowest ribs into your body on the exhales.

Beginning to inhale reach your hands up again, come back to the center.

Beginning to exhale, turn gently to the left, drawing your lowest ribs into your body. Let your hands come down, left hand behind you, right hand in front of you.

Stay here for 3 slow long even deep breaths in and out, mindful of drawing the lowest ribs into your body on the exhales.

Helpful hint: Every time we twist, the spine aligns itself and we bring fresh blood and oxygen into the internal organs. It's like getting an internal massage.

Take care to be gentle in your twists. Never yank or crank or make your body go anywhere it's not ready to go. Anne has her hand on the outside of her opposite leg. You can place your hand between your knees or on your leg. Listen to your body. Let your pelvis move as it needs and wants to.

Twist Two

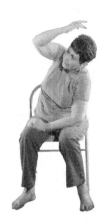

Begin in Tadasana.

Begin inhaling and reach your hands up to the sky.

Begin exhaling, walk your left foot and knee slightly forward, draw your lowest ribs into your body to be even with the top of your pelvis and turn to your right side, keeping the right hand up in the air and bringing the left forearm to the left thigh. Stretch your right hand and arm over your head. Let your pelvis move as it needs and wants to.

Breathe 3 slow long even deep breaths in and out here.

Begin inhaling and come back to the center and up.

Begin exhaling and relax your hands down.

Begin inhaling and reach your hands up to the sky.

Begin exhaling, walk your right foot and knee slightly forward, draw your lowest ribs into your body to be even with the top of your pelvis and turn to your left side, keeping the left hand up in the air and bringing the right forearm to the right thigh. Stretch your left hand and arm over your head.

Breathe 3 slow long even deep breaths in and out here.

Begin inhaling and come back to the center and up.

Begin exhaling and relax your hands down.

Twist Three

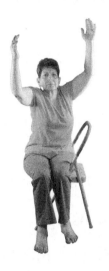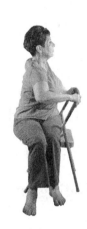

Begin in Tadasana.

Turn to your right and sit sideways in your chair.

Find Tadasana in this position.

Begin breathing in and reach your hands and arms over your head.

Begin breathing out, walk your left foot and knee slightly forward, draw your lowest ribs into your body to be even with the top of your pelvis and turn to your right so that you can place your hands on the top of the back of the chair, right hand on the right top side, left hand on the left top side. Let your left leg come even more forward if your body needs it to.

Breathe in. Breathe out drawing your lowest ribs in and using the back of the chair to support you in holding your twist. Stay here for 3 slow long even deep breaths in and out.

Begin inhaling lift arms up and come back to where you began.

Shift to the center of the chair to pause in Tadasana for a breath in and a breath out.

Turn to your left and sit sideways in your chair.

Begin inhaling and lift your arms up.

Begin exhaling walk your right foot and knee slightly forward, draw your lowest ribs into your body to be even with the top of your pelvis and turn to your left so that you can place your hands on the top of the back of the chair, right hand on the right top side, left hand on the left top side. Let your right leg come even more forward if your body needs it to.

Breathe in. Breathe out drawing your lowest ribs in and using the back of the chair to support you in holding your twist. Stay here for 3 slow long even deep breaths in and out.

Helpful hint: It's worth repeating that we want the body to guide our twist. We never want to crank or pull or push. You may notice as you relax that your body increases the twist a silly millimeter more. That's ok. But don't YOU force it!

Warrior 1 and 2
(Virabhadrasana 1 and 2)

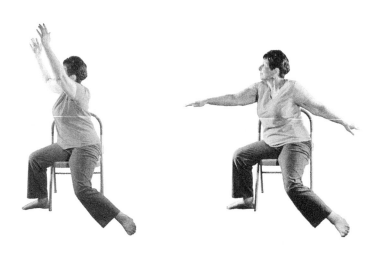

The word Virabhadrasana comes from the Sanskrit word that means courage and strength.

Just trying yoga requires your courage. In doing yoga, you exercise your courage so you can cultivate your strength, whatever strength you need—physical, emotional, spiritual, mental.

Begin in Tadasana.

Turn to your right side and point your right knee to the right.

Stretch your left leg out to the side and as far back as you comfortably can.

Begin inhaling and reach your arms up over your head. Keep looking straight ahead over your right knee.

Stay here for 3 slow long even deep breaths in and out.

When you next exhale, you can come back to Tadasana and do Virabhadrasana 1 on the other side or you can move right to Virabhadrasana 2 on the right side.

If you decide to move right to Virabhadrasana 2, from Virabhadrasana 1, turn just your upper body (mid-upper back and up) one quarter turn to the left. Bring your arms down so that they're now just below shoulder height. Reach your right finger tips away from your left finger tips and gaze over the middle finger of your right hand. Draw your lowest ribs gently into your body so they're even with the top of your pelvis.

Stay here for 3 slow long even deep breaths in and out. Remember to honor your body. If your arms get tired, let them come to your sides. Keep lifting your heart.

When you next exhale, come back to Tadasana, facing forward.

Pause here for a few breaths.

Now you can do Virabhadrasana 1 and 2 on the other side. If you choose to do Virabhadrasana 1 on the right side and then the left, and then do Virabhadrasana 2 on each side, you would start in Tadasana and do Virabhadarasana 2 on each side as well. Play with the poses!

Wide-legged Tadasana

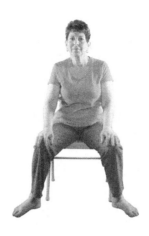

This is a great pose for relaxing the hip areas and the lower back as well. It's really important for those who sit a lot during the day and is especially valuable for people who are in a wheelchair for much of their day.

Begin in Tadasana.

Open your legs as wide as you're able. If you're using blocks under your feet, move (or have a helper move) the blocks so that they're under your feet in this new position.

You can have the block or the cushion behind you for support. And you can stay here for as long as you like, breathing slow long even deep breaths in and out.

Helpful hint: This is a great option if your hips and legs and back are too tight to do Ardha Sukhasana (half easy sitting pose or #4 pose).

"I'm not a big fan of the hip-opening poses...probably because it's what I need most."

—E, Long-time MS Yoga participant

Savasana (Final Relaxation)

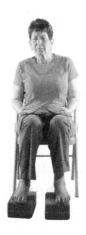

Each time we practice, we want to end in savasana or final relaxation. It gives the mind/body/spirit an opportunity to absorb and integrate all you've done. Yoga, as my teacher Judith Lasater says, is not the poses; yoga is the residue that the experience leaves on your central nervous system. Yoga leaves us feeling better than when we began. It opens our mind, our heart, and our body to changes of attitude and capacity: "Do a little yoga, change a little. Do a lot of yoga, change a lot." (Gabriel Halpern)

So please include at least 5-10 minutes of final relaxation after you've done the poses so that you may truly experience the soothing nature of yoga to your mind, body, and spirit. This can be very challenging to many people which is a sign that it's what we need!

You can choose to sit in Seated Tadasana or Wide-legged Tadasana with a block or a cushion behind you. If it's accessible to you, you may want to lie on the floor and put your legs up on the chair and a pillow under your head.

Wherever you spend your last minutes of practice, allow your breath to be your focus. Feel the breath in and out. If it helps you focus, you might count the breath: In 1 Out 1 In 2 Out 2 until 10. If you get to 10, begin again. If you don't get to 10, but instead get distracted, notice and without judging or shaming or criticizing yourself in any way, begin again.

You may want to set a gentle timer for yourself. And if 10 minutes seems not doable at first, begin with 2 minutes and gradually increase it as you're able.

All that you do, do it with love.

Some Recommended Sequences of Poses

I'm confident that when you've practiced yoga regularly for a while, you'll feel more and more comfortable doing poses as your body feels them.

In the meanwhile, I've put together the following sequences of poses so that you can begin to really enjoy your breath and flow of the poses as they meet you where you are.

If you have any questions as you learn the poses and do the sequences, please feel free to contact me at my email address: msyogawithpaula@gmail.com. I'll be happy to answer as best I can.

Sequence One
Approximately 25 Minutes

Begin in Seated Tadasana. 3-5 minutes

Become aware of your feet, your legs, your buttocks, your back, your arms and hands, your shoulders, your neck and your head.

- **Notice:** Where do you feel your breath coming into your body? your nose or your mouth

- **Notice:** Where do you feel your breath leaving your body? your nose or your mouth

- Just notice. Just breathe.

Shoulder circles.

Side stretch. Each side 3 times

Cat/cow. 5-7 repetitions

Sun Salutation 3 times.

Twist 1. 3 times each side

Twist 2. 3 times each side

Psoas softener and toner. Start by turning to your right side. Hold for up to 10-15 breaths visualizing your breath moving into and out of the space from just below your left rib cage to just above your knee cap.

Move into extended angle.

Come back to Tadasana.

Do the other side.

Wide-seated Tadasana.

Remain here for 7-10 minute Savasana breathing and being.

Sequence Two
Approximately 10-15 Minutes

Begin in Tadasana.

Feel where your breath is coming into your body. Feel where your breath is leaving your body. Notice any places in your body where you feel tense or tight and visualize your breath moving into those places, one at a time.

We'll move with the breath.

Shoulder circles 3-5 times

Sun Salutation 1 time

Twist 2

Psoas softener/toner beginning by turning to the right. Stay here and move to

Side angle

Stay on right side and move to Twist 3

Come back to Tadasana for 2 SLED breaths

Go to left side.

Psoas softener/toner then side angle then Twist 3

Come back to Tadasana.

Side Stretch

Ardha Sukhasana (#4) each side or Wide-legged Tadasana.

Tadasana for Savasana.

Sequence Three
Approximately 15-18 Minutes

Begin in Tadasana.

Scan your body from the crown of your head to the soles of your feet. Notice any tense or tight spots. Visualize your breath moving into those spaces one at a time. Become more aware of your breath and let your breath lead you in your poses.

Cat/cow 6-7 times, taking your time, moving with your SLED breaths in and out

Eagle arms 3 breaths each side

Finger/hand/shoulder release

Knot 3 breaths each side

Virabhadrasana 1 then 2 on the same side

Move to Tadasana then Virabhadrasana 1 and 2 on opposite side

Back to Tadasana.

Psoas softener/toner

Cat/cow

Top of hand stretch

Forward fold 3-5 breaths

Baddha konasana for savasana.

If this gets uncomfortable at any time, bring your feet down to the ground and come to Tadasana to complete your relaxation.

Breathing Exercises (Pranayama)

"I've learned so many things to help keep me calm and relaxed. It has helped me get through many infusion, blood tests and dental procedures.... when you find and concentrate on your breath, you can get through anything."

—AM, Longtime MS Yoga participant

While it's true that we breathe without having to think about it, it's also true that we can learn to use our breath to calm ourselves, relax ourselves, and soothe ourselves. It's also believed that the breath can be very healing.

In the yoga tradition, breathing exercises are called "pranayama." Some people call deep breathing "yoga breathing." Others call these breathing techniques. I call them practices. It doesn't matter what we call it. What's important is that we give ourselves time every day and especially in times of stress to breathe and to pay attention to our breath. And to monitor our breath throughout the day so that when we notice we're breathing shallowly (or holding our breath), we know to breathe a slow long even deep breath in and out.

Below, I share a couple of breathing practices that my students and I have found to be the most helpful.

And I invite you to what may be the most important aspect of breath work.

Receive the Breath

Awareness Comes First

One of the best ways I've found to learn breathing techniques is first to pay attention to your breath. In fact, you need to be aware in order to know what to do and then know that you're doing it!

Close your eyes and notice:

Where do you feel your breath enter your body—your nose or your mouth?

Where do you feel your breath IN your body once you breathe in—your chest? your belly? your sides? your back? All of the above? None of the above?

Where do you feel your breath leave your body—your nose or your mouth?

Which is longer—your inhale or your exhale?

Practice noticing before moving on.

In yoga, we want to breathe most of the time in and out through the nose. There are exceptions, but most of the time, this is what we aim for. The most important part, though, is to breathe! So if you have any blockage at all from a cold or any other condition that isn't allowing you to breathe through your nose, JUST BREATHE!

Following are the ways to breathe that my students find most helpful.

SLED—Slow Long Even Deep Breaths In and Out

Throughout the book, you've read "slow, long, even, deep breaths in and out." (Or SLED as I've taken to calling it...Picture a sled sliding right into relaxation!)

Place one hand on your chest and the other hand on your belly. When you breathe in, where do you feel your body expand? Most adults breathe into the chest. All of the relaxation responses (reduced heart rate, reduced respiration rate, lower blood pressure, etc. as noted by Herbert Benson and many others) are contingent on deep breathing.

Deep breathing brings your breath into your back, sides, and belly.

As you breathe in, feel the hand on your belly move out. Become aware of the sides and back of your body expanding.

As you breathe out, feel the hand on your belly move in as your belly moves in.

Breathe in—allow your back and sides and belly to move outward.

Breathe out—allow your belly sides and back to relax inward.

When my Dad was 90 years old, his doctor told him to practice yoga breathing, that is, slow long even deep breathing in and out. He found it challenging after so many years of breathing primarily in his chest. The cells of the body depend on oxygen. When we learn to breathe deeply, we bring more oxygen into the cells of our body. This creates a cascade of health.

SLED breathing at bedtime helps you relax and allows sleep to come more easily.

SLED breathing in times of stress allows your mind, body, spirit to slow down and take a step back so that you can manage whatever comes your way.

I encourage you to practice SLED breathing during yoga AND ALSO throughout your day: Every time you think of it, breathe a slow long even deep breath in and a SLOWER LONGER "EVENER" DEEPER BREATH OUT.

It's important to empty the lungs in order to make space for the fresh air to come into the lungs. Often, we breathe deeply IN but we breathe less deeply out. I invite you to breathe deeply in and even more deeply out.

Become really comfortable with SLED breathing in and out BEFORE you try the next breathing technique.

Alternate Nostril Breathing
(Nadi Shodhana)

Throughout our day, when we're healthy, we naturally alternate breathing predominantly through one nostril or the other. To tap into this naturally occurring phenomenon and help reach a state of calm, we use this natural tendency by breathing first through one nostril and then the other. (To this with me, go to my YouTube channel: https://www.youtube.com/c/MSYogaWithPaula.)

Sit in Tadasana. Use the thumb and ring finger of your right hand. Extend your index and middle fingers or bend the index and middle fingers. See which version works better for you.

Breathe in. Rest your thumb VERY gently on your right nostril where it begins to flare out from the center of the nose, rest your index and middle fingers on your forehead. Close the right nostril by GENTLY pressing your thumb against it. Leave the left nostril open and breathe out through the left nostril.

Breathe in through the left nostril. Press the ring finger VERY gently against the left nostril where it begins to flare out from the center of the nose to close it and open the right nostril. Breathe out through the right nostril.

Breathe in through the right nostril. Press the thumb gently against the right nostril to close it. Open the left nostril. Breathe out through the left nostril. Bring in through the left nostril.

Press the ring finger gently against the left nostril to close it. Open the right nostril. Breathe out through the right nostril. Breathe in through the right nostril.

Press the thumb gently against the right nostril to close it and open the left nostril. Breathe out through the left nostril. Breathe in through the left nostril. Gently press the ring finger and close the left nostril.

Open the right nostril. Breathe out through the right nostril. Breathe in through the right nostril.

Open both nostrils and breathe all the way out.

Now practice slow long even deep breathing in and out.

Savor the softness you're feeling right now.

As you become more and more comfortable and familiar with alternate nostril breathing and how it feels, you might try it now and then without using your hands and using visualization to bring the breath to each side.

REMEMBER: The most profound changes are from the simplest of things. When you do only breathing-with-awareness here and there throughout your day, you give yourself a tremendous gift.

Resources

To receive Paula Gardner's Newsletter and stay up-to-date on all things MS Chair Yoga-Related, go to https://awacbff.aweb.page/MS-Chair-Yoga and enter your name and email address. You'll receive a video you can use to practice along with me and then you'll receive all updates to Paula's programs as well as invitations to all new programs, books, yoga sequences, etc.

Beaber, M.D., Brandon. *Resilience in the Face of Multiple Sclerosis 2019*

Fishman, Loren and Small, Eric L. *Yoga and Multiple Sclerosis: A Journey to Health and Healing.* 2007: Demas Medical Publishing, LLC. New York NY

Maurer, Robert. *One Small Step Can Change Your Life: The Kaizen Way 2004,* 2014: Workman Publishing Co, Inc. New York, NY

McCall, Timothy, M.D. *Yoga as Medicine: The Yogic Prescription.* 2007: Bantam Dell, New York NY

Yoga blocks and straps are available online and in stores. I recommend Gaiam blocks and straps (available on Amazon and in sporting goods stores).

About the Author

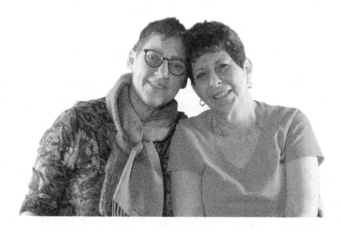

Paula Strupeck Gardner has been teaching something for 40+ years. First, it was French, English as a Second Language, Linguistics, and Methods of Teaching. She left the classroom and, after her sons were born, needing refuge, she discovered yoga. During her first-ever savasana, Paula KNEW that she wanted to bring this feeling of ease and peace to everyone.

After getting certified as a yoga teacher, Paula began working with people—seniors and a group of folks with Multiple Sclerosis—who couldn't do "regular" yoga. She adapted the poses to their bodies and began using a chair for support. This quickly evolved into "chair yoga" where the participants sat to do the poses, stood for some of the poses (because we need to keep our legs as strong as we're able!) and relaxed at the end of the practice in their chair.

When she began, no certifications existed in yoga for people with MS. Paula sought out information from MS organizations to learn more about the disease and about general exercise programs for MS. Paula is deeply indebted to Joy Wagner, creator of fitMS and founder of NeuroBalance Center (https://neurobalancecenter.org/)of Barrington IL for her help in understanding how MS ravages the body/mind/spirit and for inspiring her to incorporate yoga into the fitness program at Orland Park Health and Fitness. Paula has also learned a great deal from her students who have shared their stories with deep honesty.

A perennial student, Paula has continued to learn and grow in her practice and study of yoga, meditation, and ayurveda so that she can support you in your desire to integrate yoga, ayurveda and/or meditation into YOUR life.

She regularly teaches Chair Yoga in person and online to students from around the world and is especially devoted to bringing yoga to people with MS, Parkinson's, Fibromyalgia, COPD, myasthenia gravis, and other conditions that make it challenging to participate in yoga outside their home.

Paula welcomes you to join her mission to do yoga for the rest of your life. You can stay in touch with Paula by subscribing to her email (https://awacbff.aweb. page/MS-Chair-Yoga). You'll receive a free video so you can practice with Paula and you'll be notified of all online and in-person events as well as receive guided meditations and other helpful tools.

Paula lives with her husband of 30 years in a Chicago suburb. Their sons, who Paula describes as "the lights of my life; my gurus" are grown and making their lives in music and the writing arts. She counts yoga as one of the greatest blessings of her life. And looks forward to sharing it with you.

About the Model

Anne Matty was diagnosed with Relapsing Remitting Multiple Sclerosis in 1987 when her sons were 7 and 8 years old. She experienced several hospitalizations for steroid treatments for flare ups before beginning medication to modify the disease.

She has stayed as active as MS has allowed: In 2002, she was among the first members of the then newly formed MS Aquatics Program at what was called Palos Health and Fitness Center and is now Orland Park Health and Fitness Center. Anne describes it as being one of the best things she's ever done!

A year later, when Paula Gardner added yoga to the MS program, Anne found that what she practiced in yoga translated to her entire life—She found herself practicing stretches throughout her day, standing tall with alignment, and noticed that her "yoga breathing" helped her stay more comfortable through infusions, blood draws, dental works and life's little aggravations.

After Anne broke her arm in 2008 and was in a cast for three months, she found that it wasn't until she was back to yoga that she regained most of the mobility she had lost.

In 2019, Chicago's WGN TV featured Anne in its show, Living Healthy Chicago, where she demonstrated and discussed her experience living and keeping healthy with MS. You can watch it at https://www.youtube.com/watch?v=3wrWudX9Kh0! Anne has also been featured in a promotional video for the Neurology Department's MS Clinic of Loyola University's Medical Center.

Anne and her husband Ray have been married for 43 years and have six grandchildren whom they adore! They live in the Chicago area.

Anne is grateful to yoga not only for the calmness, stretching and strength she feels has come from yoga, but also for her cherished friendship with Paula. "I encourage all of you to not only try yoga, but to do it for the rest of your life."

How Can You Help?

Thank you for allowing me to help you take excellent care of yourself! Please do me the kindness of leaving your honest review so that others can see how this book has helped you bring yoga to you in YOUR home.

I am donating 20% of the net profits of this to the MS Society, MS Focus, and other local MS groups.

If you'd like to donate directly to a particular organization, please go to the website of the organization(s) you choose to support. Their web addresses are listed below:

MS Society's South Cook Self-Help Group
(https://bit.ly/32DOgcW)
We thank you for your support!

MS Focus
https://msfocus.org/MS-Chair-Yoga-At-Home.aspx

Working on Wellness Foundation
https://www.workingonwellnessfoundation.org/

I'd love to hear YOUR story. If you have also written a book or would like to share YOUR story, get more information from Self-Publishing School by going to their site (https://self-publishingschool.com/refer/). I've found them to be extraordinarily helpful as I navigated writing and publishing this book. I'm certain you'll have the same experience. And your story is worth telling and reading!

Many Blessings Always,

Made in the USA
Las Vegas, NV
06 December 2023

82032176R00066